RESISTANCE BAND WORKOUT FOR SENIORS

A QUICK AND CONVENIENT SOLUTION FOR SENIOR MEN AND WOMEN TO MOVE THEIR BODIES, IMPROVE THEIR STRENGTH, AND OVERALL HEALTH WHILE AT HOME

FIT FOREVER

CONTENTS

YOUR FIRST STEPS

We have always been told that working out and staying active is an important part of maintaining one's physical health, which not only impacts how we look, but our physical and mental health and overall mood. However, staying fit is not always easy. Going to the gym requires travel time, a membership cost, sharing equipment with other gym-goers, and sometimes the fear of being judged by others. Using equipment like weights or a treadmill also makes it harder to continue your regular workout routine when traveling. In some cases, high-impact workouts like using weights or jumping around can hurt your joints after an extended period of time.

As a senior, you have maintained your physique and have a deep connection with your body that you have developed over the years. You have probably tried multiple forms of exercise, and learned what is or is not effective for you, your lifestyle, and your needs. Whether you are tired of trying new routines or know what does and doesn't work for you, you are in the right place to learn about a very favorable form of movement.

An easy and convenient exercise that can be modified to create a new routine, while always offering modifications for different levels, is resistance band training. Sometimes, resistance band training is overlooked because workout equipment like weights or treadmills are more common within a gym. However, resistance band training offers a variety of benefits that are just as helpful as any other workout, while being more convenient.

Through your decision to begin this specific type of workout regime, you are opening the door for you to be able to work out, strengthen, and improve your health in the comfort of your home, at any point of the day, and through very little cost. You are making a great choice in your health journey, and over time will see the benefits of resistance training. The ability to workout at home, at any point of the day, and with a therapy band will prove to you that working out does not, and should not, be a hassle.

As your workouts become easier and you become stronger, you will be grateful for the day you opened this book and grabbed your resistance band. You have already made the first big step in creating a more effective physical exercise plan by dedicating your time and effort to learn about the benefits of this specific training. You are already doing great, and should maintain both focus and motivation to continue your progress towards a healthy and convenient lifestyle. So get ready to start moving, and follow along in an easy-to-comprehend guide to gain control over a new workout routine.

1

IMPORTANCE OF RESISTANCE BAND TRAINING

Like any other type of physical activity, resistance training comes with its own set of benefits and results. Resistance training is used for a number of reasons, and when used properly, its benefits have an increasingly positive effect on the individual. But before we begin, let's refine and clarify what resistance training actually is.

Resistance training is a specific type of workout in which the individual uses a resistance (either with the band or weights) to perform simple movements acting like a pulling system against a force that resists the movement to gain strength, flexibility, and endurance for the targeted muscle group. Resistance bands are a common tool used in resistance training and are a flexible material that can be stretched and returned to the original shape in one movement. Unlike weight training, resistance bands are good for seniors to refine their strength, rather than pushing their bodies past their limits with weights that are too heavy for them to handle properly at home.

The most easily identifiable benefits of resistance training are that it can be done anywhere, and the only materials needed are the resistance band. In addition, because resistance band training can be done at home, you don't have to go to the gym to workout. The convenience and simplicity of the band allow the user to exercise on their time, at their pace, and in the comfort of their homes.

Resistance bands themselves are cheap, typically have a long lifespan when taken care of, and come in a variety of sizes and strengths. They are easy to pack, lightweight, and versatile for when you travel. One band can be used for multiple exercises. As you will soon discover, the band can be tied to a sturdy structure, wrapped around your body, or used freely without additional support.

The physical benefits of resistance bands include the fact that it reduces body fat, like most other exercises, while incorporating flexibility, strength, and aerobics. It can also decrease heavy cardiovascular demand found in other cardio workouts, increase balance and stability, and stretch in a way that is both manageable and challenging.

Lastly, the greatest use of resistance band training for seniors is that the exercises are versatile and can be adjusted to accommodate your specific needs. If you are starting resistance band workouts for the first time, or need an easier workout day, then you have the option to either lower the number of repetitions and sets, or use a lighter band. If you are feeling great one day and would like to challenge yourself, then you can make adjustments by using a stronger band or increasing repetitions. Alternatively, some of these exercises could be used without a band to ensure proper alignment before adding the resistance.

RESISTANCE TRAINING IN ATHLETES

Many athletes use resistance bands for the same reasons that you might use them. Although a professional athlete does more in a day than just band exercises, they use a combination of band, weight, and aerobics to complement each other and create a routine that leaves them in peak physical condition. Band training is used on peak performance days, daily drills, and for rehabilitation after an injury.

Even though you may not train like a professional athlete (or maybe you do), you can learn from their training regime and use their tips. In most cases, athletes use resistance band training as a form of injury recovery and prevention. Physical therapists administer resistance band exercises to strengthen and isolate a specific point of the body to increase mobility, agility, and strength. In essence, resistance band training offers plenty of results when used properly.

The use of the band allows for resistance training without placing the same amount of pressure on the joints as weights do, which creates a decrease in the amount of post-workout inflammation. These are great examples of why resistance can be a great opportunity for you; because your workouts will be performed either at home or in a private area, you want to increase injury prevention, while allowing yourself to feel great, free of inflammation after a workout that you performed alone.

In general, athletes use resistance band exercises to warm up for a long day of physical activity because the results allow them to maintain their physique, train specific muscle groups in a safe, low-impact movement, stretch and strengthening workout. Sometimes, athletes have a few bands that they switch out based on the amount of resistance, length, or shape of the band they need or want for a specific exercise. The options to use and modify band exercises are endless, and the benefits of the workout are seen in both athletes and seniors alike.

2

TYPES OF RESISTANCE BANDS

The range of exercises, paired with the different variety of levels of people who use resistance training, means that there are so many options of resistance bands available to you. It's important for you to choose a band that compliments your workout based on the band shape, size, and strength.

The resistance band is typically a piece of material, made of a flexible elastic so that it can be stretched and returned to its original shape. The elasticity allows you to use resistance in a movement so that your muscles contract to avoid jerking motions, or can assist you in a stretch by pulling you in a certain direction. The production of shape, size, and strength of the bands vary.

Firstly, the strength of the band that you get will depend on your comfort levels in the exercises. It's generally recommended to start with a band that is lighter in strength, then build your way onto a stronger band as you become more stable and precise in the movements. Just like weights, using a band that you are not ready for can be dangerous, since it is still a resistance tool. A heavy strength band will be stronger, while a lighter band will offer less resistance to your movements. The strength levels of the band vary based on the company or brand that you buy it from. Some bands come in packs of light, medium, and heavy resistance, while others offer even more strength variety. Most brands color coordinate their levels of strength so that you know which band you are reaching for with a quick glance. The colors vary based on the brand, and you can easily find the spectrum by checking the box.

Next, the size of the band plays a role in the types of exercises you can do with it. For example, you will notice that some exercises require a longer band to wrap it around your body, pull it from an anchored point, or stretch the length of your wingspan and height. In contrast, other exercises only need the band to wrap around your two legs. However, an added benefit of the elasticity found in most bands is that they can easily be cut with a simple pair of scissors if your band is too long for you. Just keep in mind that you can always cut more, but would have to purchase a new band if you cut too short.

The shape of your band is more of a personal choice than a recommendation. The most common and versatile band is a simple length of elastic material. With this therapy band, you are able to tie it, wrap it, cut it, and perform any of these exercises listed in the upcoming chapters and more. Next, a mini loop band is made to be like an oversized rubber band, and removes the step of having to tie and untie a therapy band. These are often smaller in size, and limit your ability to perform some exercises. Lastly, a tube band resembles a jump rope, but the elasticity of the tube band allows you to use it in these exercises. In some bands, the ends shape into handles, making it easier to hold when you have to stretch the band.

Due to the elasticity of the band, proper care is essential to ensure a long lifespan. Resistance bands can last a while, but you must watch out for wear and tear to ensure that it doesn't break mid-stretch. Be on the lookout for small tears, or loss of durability in the elastic. If the band begins to feel lighter, then the chances of it breaking while you are using it becomes higher. Keep your band away from direct sunlight and sticky substances. You can easily store your bands by folding them and setting them in a container.

You can find resistance bands most anywhere that sells workout equipment, both in physical stores and online. Different brands or makers will offer different options in strength, size, color coordination, and shape, so it's best to understand which options you would prefer to use before going resistance band shopping.

RECOMMENDED

Because of the variety of bands, knowing where to start and what you want in a band is a good idea before you purchase one. Think about the styles of bands, from strength to size.

For the first time trying new exercises, or resistance bands in general, it is recommended to start with a lighter band to ensure that you are using proper form and activating the correct muscles to prevent any injuries. As you become more comfortable in the movements and feel like the exercises are becoming easier, then you can advance to an intermediate strength band. Keep in mind that different parts of the body are stronger than others, so you may use a lighter band on your arms than you do legs. When you feel yourself progressing and advancing in these exercises, having different band strengths can become a good way to keep your workout routine dynamic.

The shape and length of your band is up to you. The most versatile band that works for all of the following exercises would be a longer band, about your height, without the end handles. However, if you find yourself struggling with excess bad in some exercises, or become tired of tying the band to create loops, then having a variety of band styles is a good option for you.

3

HOW TO CREATE AN EFFECTIVE WORKOUT ROUTINE

To begin creating an effective workout, you must first understand your level of fitness. This will depend on the number of days you workout in a week, the intensity of your workout, your diet, age, and any medical conditions.

A beginner level works out about two to three days a week, usually in about 30-minute increments. These workouts focus on low impact and intensity levels, using a lower amount of repetitions and sets, and a lighter band strength.

Intermediate levels workout three to four days in one week, typically following a 30-60 minute workout routine. These workouts increase the impact, and intensity by raising the number of repetitions and sets while using a medium-strength band.

An advanced level works out four to six days per week at 40-90 minute workout routines. These regimes follow the highest impact and most intense structures. They incorporate impact and intensity by maximizing the number of repetitions, sets, and band strength.

The key to a safe yet challenging workout is in the preparation. Know what you want to do, your physical limits, and your goals. Create a weekly routine that benefits your specific needs. For example, an intermediate level may workout arms on day one, legs on day two, back and core on day three, and chest and shoulders on day four, implementing rest days between workouts. Choosing what specific exercises you want to do on each day is up to you, but be sure to work each part of the body equally.

Don't forget that an essential part of the exercise is rest and recovery. As much as we may think that exercise is all about the push, you have to also know when to stop and let your body take in everything you just asked it to do. Eat a balanced diet and stay hydrated before and after rigorous workouts. Be sure to get enough sleep and exercise when you are ready.

To maintain focus and motivation, try to workout at a specific time or create a dedicated space in your home to workout in. When you keep up a strict routine, you are less likely to skip a day, or avoid using your band. Decorate your workout area with motivating quotes, pictures of your goals, or anything that makes you want to exercise.

REPETITIONS

Creating an effective workout takes the next step when you decide on the correct amount of repetitions and sets for each exercise. Repetitions of an exercise is the number of times that you repeat one movement, or exercise. The number of sets that you do is the number of times you repeat each group of repetitions. For example, you may repeat a bicep curl ten times. The number ten is the number of times you repeat the movement, or the repetitions. After ten bicep curls, you take a short break, then do another ten repetitions. This equates to two sets.

Once again, these decisions of repetitions and sets depend on your personal goals. If you want to target strength within the muscles, then you should increase the number of sets you do. However, to train proper alignment and activation of the muscle, then you would lower the number of repetitions and sets and take the exercise slowly, and focus on your body awareness. Lastly, if endurance is your goal, then the ideal choice is to increase the number of repetitions and take shorter breaks between sets.

For a normal, intermediate workout, you should start with five to ten repetitions, and three sets. Some exercises will vary depending on your initial strength, endurance, or proper alignment of your body. Make sure that you never sacrifice your safety, or quality of workout for the sake of completing your goals. Don't forget to repeat each exercise on both sides, if applicable, and to keep your workouts well-rounded, meaning that you don't skip a muscle group for any reason. Use each exercise as equally as the next.

QUALITY OVER QUANTITY

In order to ensure proper use of these exercises, keep in mind a few key tips.

Firstly, because the key aspect of resistance bands is to resist your movements, you should be working against the band. In each position, make sure that the band slightly resists your positions and movement. When you feel that the exercises become easier, then you can create a tighter resistance or move onto a stronger band.

Make sure that you are doing each exercise properly and safely, which is important as we should protect our bodies, especially at home, without a professional watching over us. To do this, follow directions slowly and accurately, and only move your body as directed. Additional movements in the body that aren't specifically instructed can lead to injuries like strains, improper twisting, or using the wrong muscles to do the movement.

If you find yourself wiggling or moving more than instructed, try the beginner suggestions and use your body awareness to check that you are activating the correct muscle groups. Only move as far as you can physically go without sacrificing your form. Be sure to move slowly and avoid any jerking motions. When you jerk in your movements, then you are either unable to support your movements with your strength, moving past your limits, or letting the band control you rather than you controlling the band.

Once you find yourself performing each exercise smoothly and are able to do so without additional movement, pause as the height of the movement where the targeted muscle is most activated. In doing this, you are giving your muscles a chance to feel the activation, improving your muscle memory and building more strength. However, if there is any extra pain like cramps or sharp pain, always listen to your body. You know what does or does not feel right because you are the one that is most in tune with how you feel.

During your resistance band exercises, you may be asked to hold the band in your hands. To ensure that the ends of the band don't slip, try wrapping the ends around your palms and holding the excess by making fists. Any time you have to wrap the band around your body, be careful not to wrap too tightly, since the elasticity of the band can become harmful.

When using your band, to avoid it snapping back on you, keep a relatively tight resistance, while also allowing some room for a range of movement. When wrapping, anchoring, or holding the band, make sure that it is secure and stable. Taking one extra precautionary step will decrease your chances of small inconveniences like having to reset each exercise between sets. Holding your band too tightly, or stretching it too far can cause the band to either snap back onto you or create small tears that can lead to it eventually breaking.

Lastly, protect yourself with good quality workout equipment, like supportive shoes. The more you are on your feet, including exercises, the more you should ensure that your feet are protected because they also support your back, preventing you from future injury.

In addition, you can also invest in a good yoga mat, since some of these exercises rely on you laying on the floor. Using the mat also provides an additional cushion between you and the hard floor, which protects your joints further.

4

THE WORKOUT

While doing the actual exercises is the fun part of trying a new workout routine, you should always prepare each workout routine with a short, yet effective warm-up. Warming up is an essential key in any workout because it sets you in the right mindset to workout, and prevents injuries by slowly introducing your body to movements and raising your heart rate. What's important is that you walk before you run.

Start a workout by warming up with cardio, which is effective in pumping your blood before using any strength-based exercises. Cardio does not always have to be running at high speed, but it can also be a brisk walk, a dance-based class, or using the elliptical or bike if that is available to you. The warmup routine you choose is up to you and based on what you have available at any given point in time.

Beginner warmup: Circle your arms forward for 30 seconds, then backward for 30 seconds, then jog in place or speed-walk for 30 seconds. Take a one-minute rest, then repeat.

Intermediate warmup: Squat 10 times, followed by a 30-second jog. Take a one-minute rest, then repeat.

Advanced warmup: Jog in place for one minute, followed by 30 seconds of jumping jacks. Take a one-minute rest, then repeat.

Once you have completed your warmup, then you can move onto strength-based exercises, such as your resistance band exercises. Now that your blood is pumping, you have raised your heart rate to a proper BPM, and your muscles have been loosened up, strength training is more likely to have a better impact on your body. You will find the exercises below, sorted by different muscle groups.

A great way to complete your workout is by stretching. The cool-down part of your workout is just as important as any other steps because it brings your body temperature and heart rate back down to normal. When cooling down, stretching is a great way to relax and improve your flexibility. Stretching is more useful after a workout because your muscles are warmer, meaning they are more likely to stretch than when they are cold. This form of cooldown also allows you to release any tension that could have been built up during the workout.

Of course, rest and recovery is another important aspect of working out. After a heavy workout, make sure that you are hydrated, eat enough, and take a proper amount of rest between workouts.

Now, you are ready to start learning the exercises that will improve your strength both conveniently and beneficially.

ARMS

1.) Curls

Band: Long band, either with handles, a tube, or a therapy band.

Step 1: Stand with feet shoulder-width apart on top of the middle of the band with a straight back holding the ends of the band in both hands, palms facing away from your body.

Step 2: Bend your elbows and bring your palms upwards to your shoulder and lower back down, then return to the original position.

Beginner: Use a lighter band, or hold the band closer to the ends. You can also opt for bodyweight, rather than using a band.

Advanced: Use a stronger band, or hold the band closer to the middle, which increases resistance.

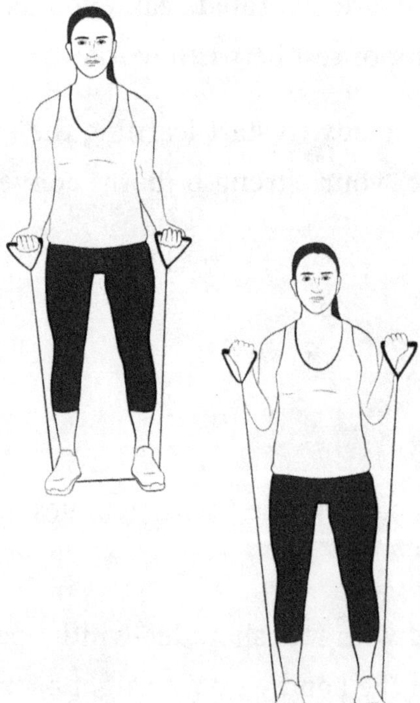

2.) Concentration curl

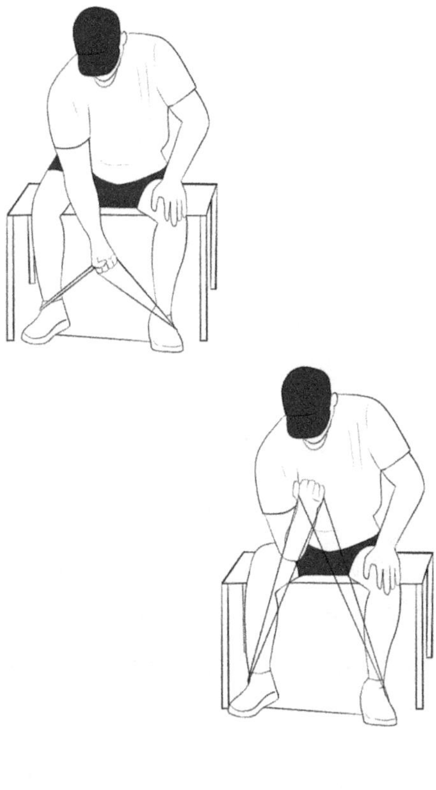

Band: Medium-sized band, either looped, with handles, a tube, or a therapy band.

Step 1: Sitting in a chair, place one foot over one end of the band, and the other foot over the middle of the band. Hold the free end of the band on the opposite side in your hand, so that the band crosses over your leg. Lean forward to place that elbow on the inside of your thigh.

Step 2: Bend at the elbow to bring your hand to your shoulder, then return to the original position.

Beginner: Use a lighter band, or hold closer to the end to create less resistance.

Advanced: Create more resistance by holding the band closer to the middle, or use a stronger band.

3.) Tricep kickbacks

Band: Medium-sized band, either with handles, a tube, or a therapy band.

Step 1: Stand with feet shoulder-width apart on top of the middle of the band with a bend in the hips so that your back creates a diagonal line, holding the ends of the band, palms facing your body.

Step 2: Extend your arms behind you in line with your back, then bend at the elbows to bring your palms towards your shoulder, then return to the original position.

Beginner: Use a lighter band or just your bodyweight. You can also hold closer to the ends.

Advanced: Bend more at the hips to create a steeper diagonal line, or use a stronger band.

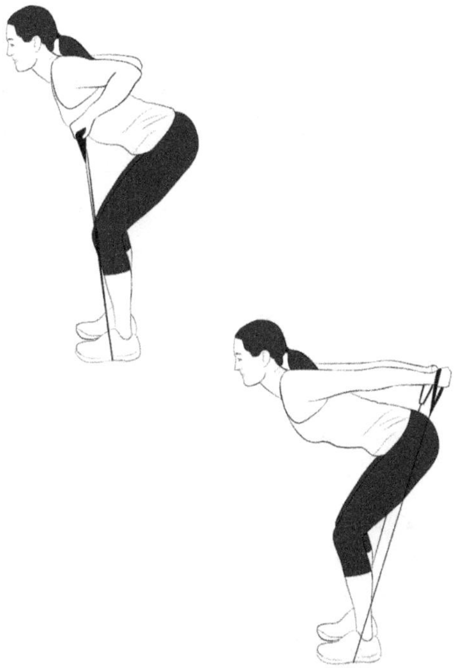

4.) Open and close

Band: Long band, either with handles, tube, or a therapy band.

Step 1: Stand with feet shoulder-width apart with a straight back, holding the band in each hand, shoulder-width apart in front of your chest, and palms face down.

Step 2: Open your arms away from each other to extend the band, then bring it back to the original position.

Beginner: Open your arms less, creating a 45 degree from your starting point, or use a lighter band.

Advanced: Open your arms to reach your sides, pausing for a moment before you close. You may also hold the band closer to the middle.

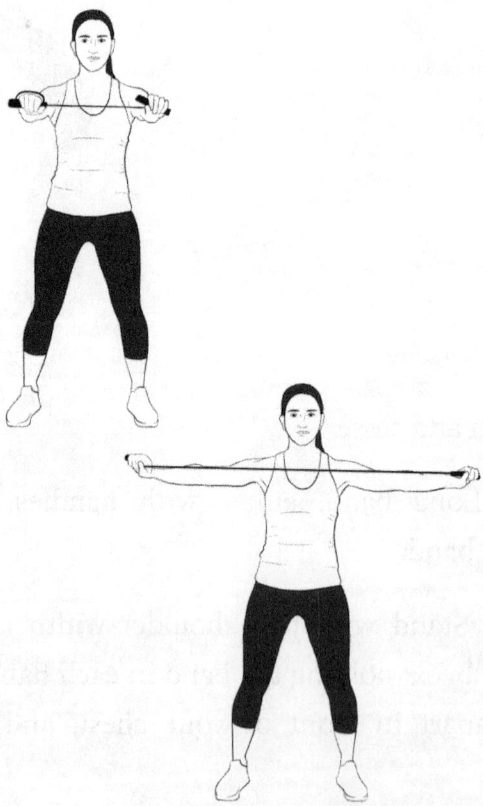

5.) Overhead triceps extension

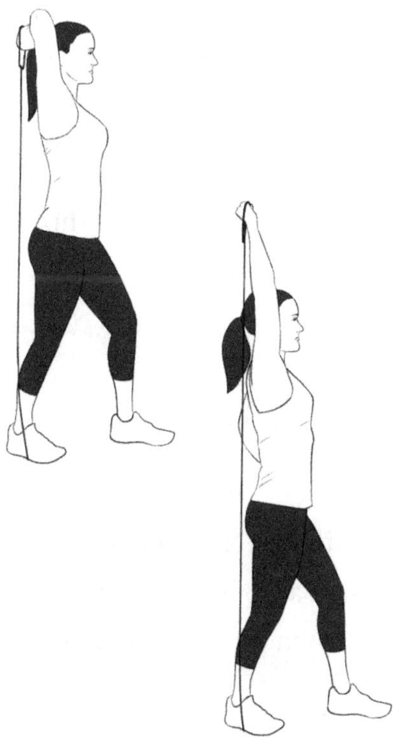

Band: Long band, either with handles, tube, or a therapy band.

Step 1: Stand with your feet in a staggered position and a straight back over one end of the band. Hold the other end of the band in both hands, behind your upper back, with bent elbows reaching towards the ceiling.

Step 2: Extend your arms and reach your hands towards the ceiling, then return to the original position.

Beginner: Use a lighter band, your own body weight, or hold the band at the ends. Alter the original position to sitting if this works better for you by sitting on the band and completing the rest of the exercise as normal.

Advanced: Use a stronger band, or hold it closer to the middle rather than the ends.

6.) Wide curls

Band: Long band, either with handles, a tube, or a therapy band.

Step 1: Stand with feet shoulder-width apart on top of the middle of the band, holding the ends in both hands, arms extended down and palms facing away from your sides.

Step 2: Keeping your elbows at your torso, bend at the elbow to lift your palms to the corresponding shoulders. Return to the original position.

Beginner: Use your own bodyweight, or a lighter band. Alternate arms instead of doing both at the same time.

Advanced: Use a stronger band or hold the band closer to the middle.

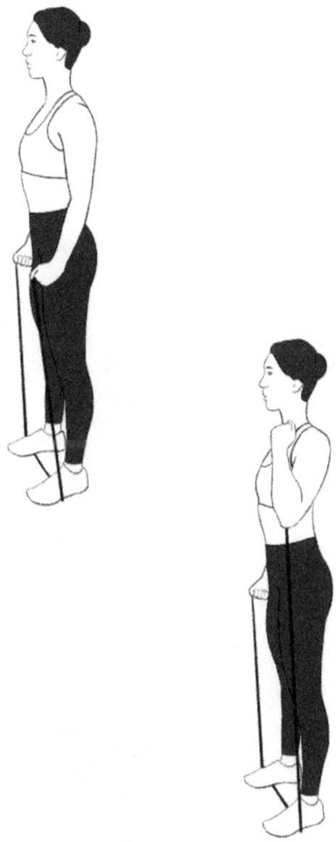

LEGS

7.) Clamshells

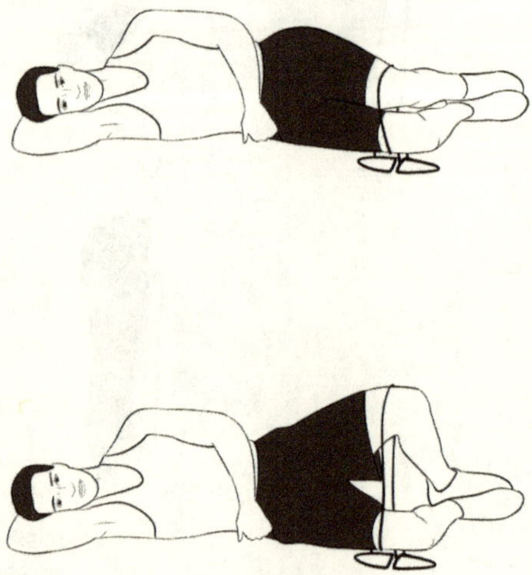

Band: Short band, either looped or a therapy band looped.

Step 1: Tie the band together to create a loop that your legs can fit through. Laying on your back, place the band to hold your legs closed together above the knee with your feet on the floor and knees pointed towards the ceiling.

Step 2: Open your knees apart and slowly return to the original position.

Beginner: Use just your body weight, a larger loop, or a lighter band. Moving the band further from your knees creates less resistance.

Advanced: Use a stronger band or a smaller loop. Move the band closer to your knees for more resistance.

8.) Squats

Band: Long band, either with handles, tube, or a therapy band.

Step 1: Stand with feet shoulder-width apart on top of the middle of the band, holding the ends of the band in both hands, palms on top of your shoulders, elbows pointing forward.

Step 2: Bend your knees slightly and lean forward, as if you were about to sit in a chair and return to the original position.

Beginner: Don't bend the knees too far; use a lighter band, or just your bodyweight.

Advanced: Bend further down, use a stronger band, or hold the band closer to the middle to create more resistance.

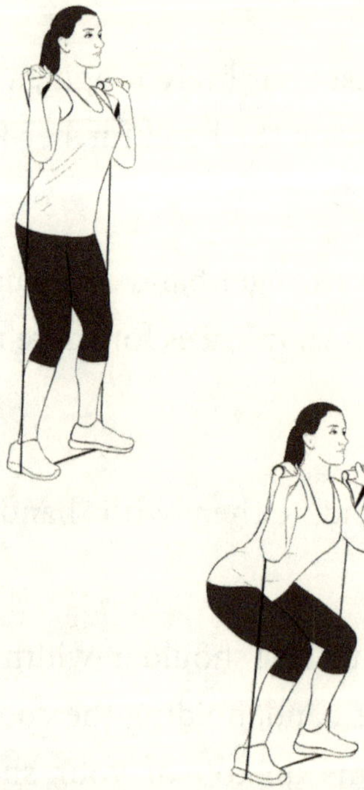

9.) Leg extension

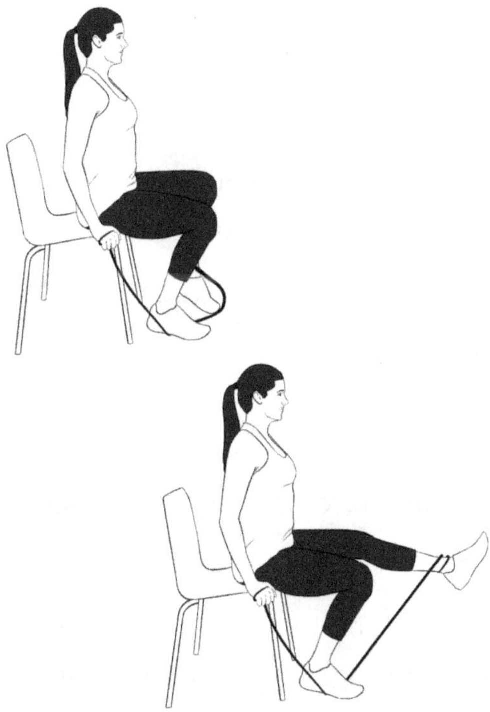

Band: Medium-sized band, either looped or a therapy band looped.

Step 1: Tie the band together to create a loop that your ankle can fit through. Sitting down over an edge, hold the band in one hand and anchor it to the ground with the foot of the chair with the loop around your ankle of the same hand the band is in.

Step 2: Extend the leg that the band is on so that it is straight, parallel to the floor, then return to the original position.

Beginner: Use just your bodyweight, or a larger loop. You don't have to extend your leg fully.

Advanced: Use a smaller loop, extending your leg completely.

10.) Leg curls

Band: Medium-sized band, either looped or a therapy band looped.

Step 1: Tie the band together to create a loop that your ankle can fit through. Laying on your stomach, anchor the loop around a stable object, like a heavy chair or bed frame, and loop the other end around your ankle.

Step 2: Bending at the knee, pull your heel towards your back as far as you can, and return to the original position.

Beginner: Don't reach your heel all the way towards your body, or use just your bodyweight.

Advanced: Bend the knee fully, or use a smaller loop.

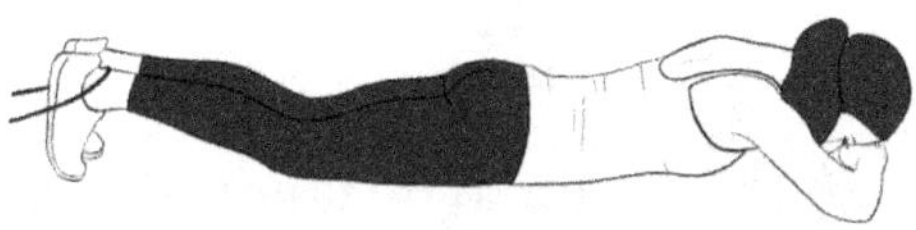

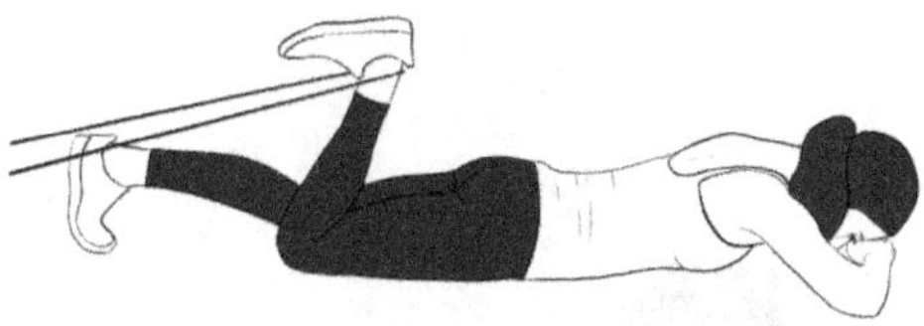

11.) Standing adduction

Band: Short band, either looped or a therapy band looped.

Step 1: Tie the band together to create a loop that your ankle can fit through.

Step 2: Place both feet within the band at ankle height, and stand with a straight back, feet shoulder-width apart. Lift one leg out to the side, keeping a straight leg, and return to the original position.

Beginner: Lift the leg two to three inches off the ground.

Advanced: Lift the leg up to one foot off the ground.

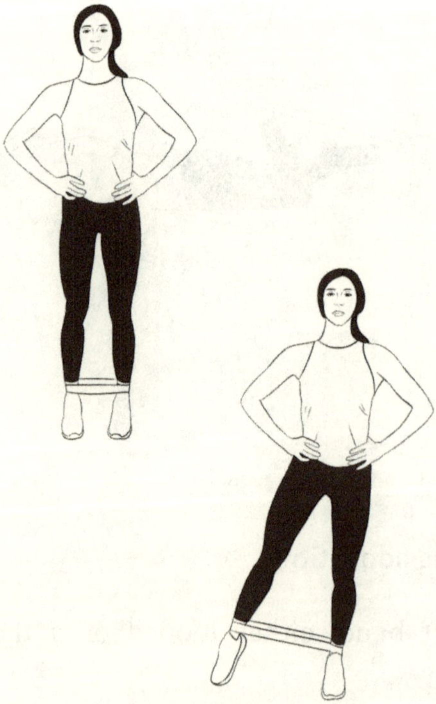

12.) Ankle stability

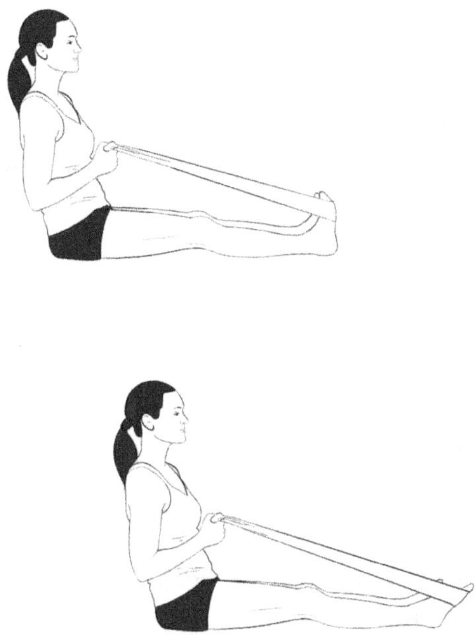

Band: Medium-sized, therapy band.

Step 1: Sitting with your legs straight in front of you, loop the band around the underside of the feet and hold the ends of the band on one or both hands.

Step 2: Point your toes towards the ground, holding the ankles together, then flex your feet, so your toes point towards the ceiling.

Beginner: Ditch the band.

Advanced: Move your feet slowly, like a wave. Point the tip of the toes last and flex the tips of the toes first.

CHEST

13.) Lower chest flye

Band: A long band with handles, a tube, or a therapy band.

Step 1: Stand in a lunge position with the back foot over the middle of the band and a straight back. Hold the ends on the band in both hands, arms extended straight down, palms facing away from your body.

Step 2: Keeping your arms straight, move your palms towards each other in front of your chest. Return to the original position.

Beginner: Use a lighter band or your bodyweight.

Advanced: Use a stronger band or hold the band closer to the middle. Bend the front knee to create a deeper lunge.

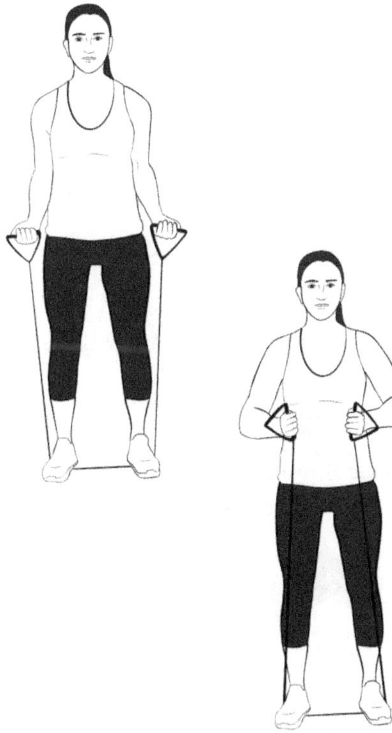

14.) Resistance chest press

Band: Long band, either a tube or a therapy band.

Step 1: Anchor the middle of the band to a stable object like a doorframe behind you at about your height. While standing in a lunge position, hold the ends of the band with both hands, palms at your chest and facing down, elbows bent and facing the sides.

Step 2: Straighten your arms in front of you, and return to the original position.

Beginner: Use a lighter band, and don't worry about fully extending your arms.

Advanced: Use a stronger band or hold closer to the middle to create more resistance.

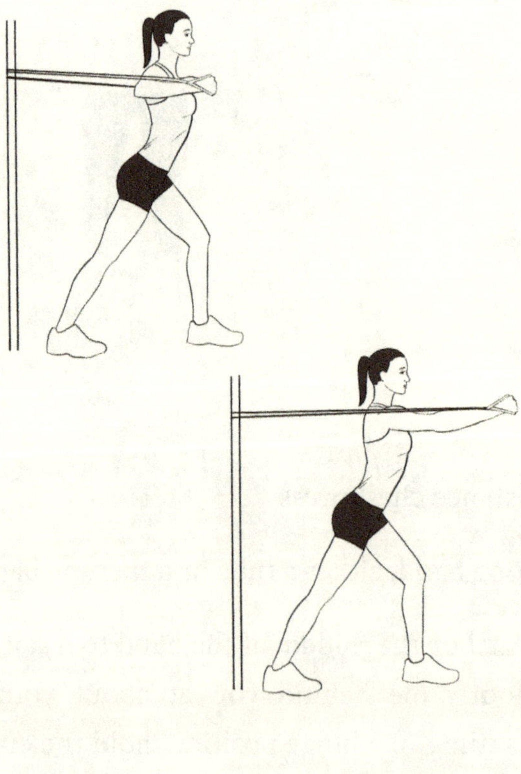

15.) Flye

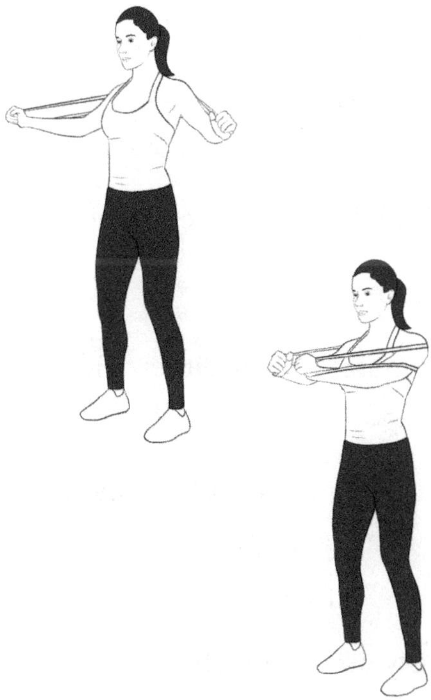

Band: Long band, either with handles, a tube, or a therapy band.

Step 1: Wrapping the band around your upper back, hold the ends of the band with both hands, standing with a straight back, arms extended to the side, and palms facing forward.

Step 2: Move your hands to the front of you, keeping the elbows straight, then return to the original position.

Beginner: Use just your bodyweight. You can also modify it to sit down.

Advanced: Hold the band closer to the middle.

16.) Resistance bench press

Band: Medium-sized band, either with handles, a tube or a therapy band.

Step 1: Anchor the middle of the band to the underside of the bench, lying face up, hold the ends of the band in both hands, elbows pointing away from your body.

Step 2: Place your hands above your shoulders, and move your arms in an upward motion like you are punching the ceiling, return to the original position.

Beginner: Use just your bodyweight or a light band. Alternate arms instead of using both if you tire easily.

Advanced: Use a stringer band, or hold closer to the middle.

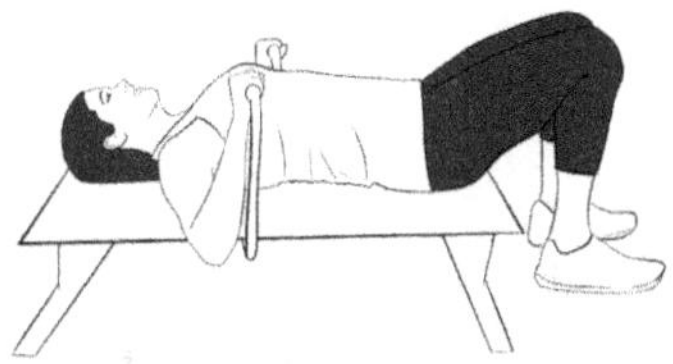

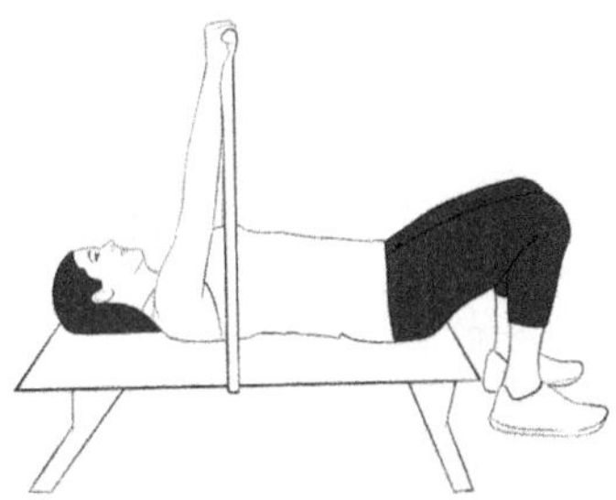

17.) Resistance push up

Band: Medium-sized band, either a tube or a therapy band.

Step 1: Wrapping the band around your upper back, hold the ends of the band with both hands, and support yourself in a plank position by placing your hands and feet on the floor and keeping your torso straight.

Step 2: Bend at the elbows, lowering your body to the ground in one position, and straighten your arms to return to the original position.

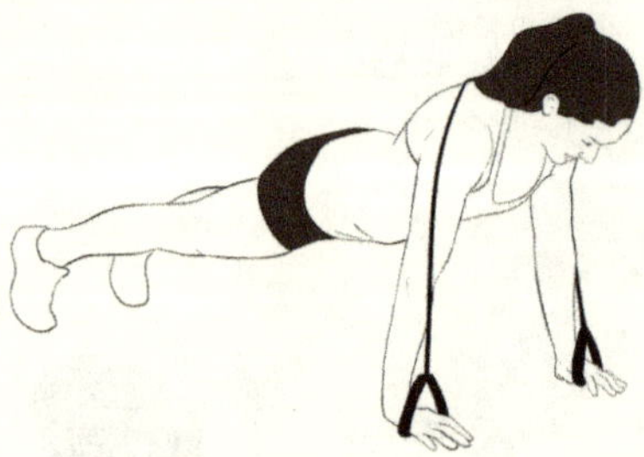

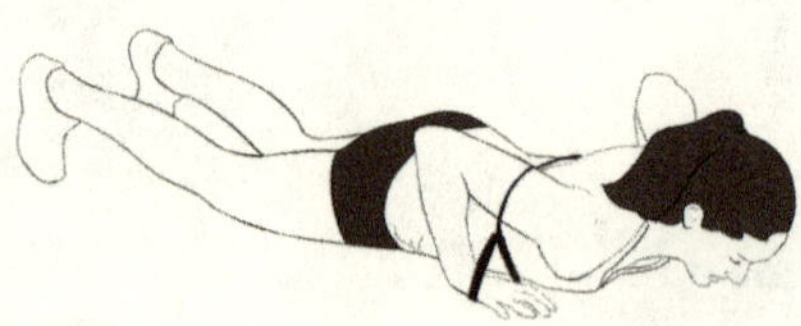

Beginner: Push up against a wall instead of on the ground, or use your bodyweight instead of a band either standing or planking.

Advanced: Hold the band closer to the middle to create more resistance in the push-up. Try different push-up variations.

SHOULDERS

18.) Overhead press

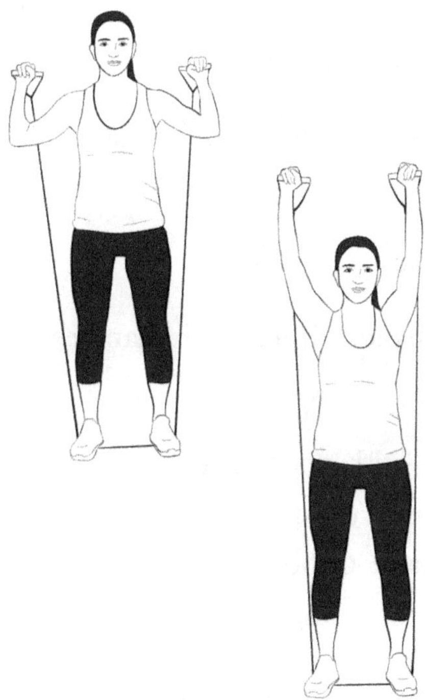

Band: Long band, either with handles, a tube, or a therapy band.

Step 1: Stand with a straight back and feet shoulder-width apart over the middle of the band holding the ends of the band in both hands. Place your hands on your shoulders, palms facing away from your body.

Step 2: Extend your arms upward as if you were punching the ceiling. Return to the original position.

Beginner: Use your bodyweight or a lighter band. Modify to a sitting position.

Advanced: Use a stronger band or hold the band closer to the middle.

19.) Forward raise

Band: Long band, either with handles, a tube, or a therapy band.

Step 1: Stand with a straight back and feet shoulder-width apart over the middle of the band holding the ends of the band in both hands. Place your hands by your sides, palms facing behind you.

Step 2: Keeping your arms extended, reach your hands forward until they lift to chest height, still straight. Return to the original position.

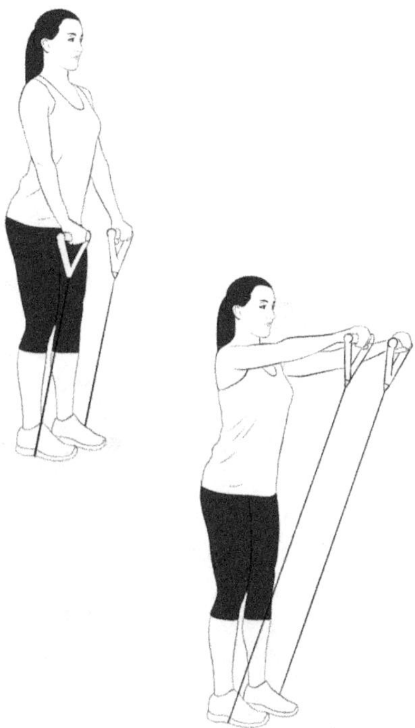

Beginner: Use just your bodyweight or a lighter band.

Advanced: Use a stronger band or hold the band closer to the middle.

20.) Lateral raise

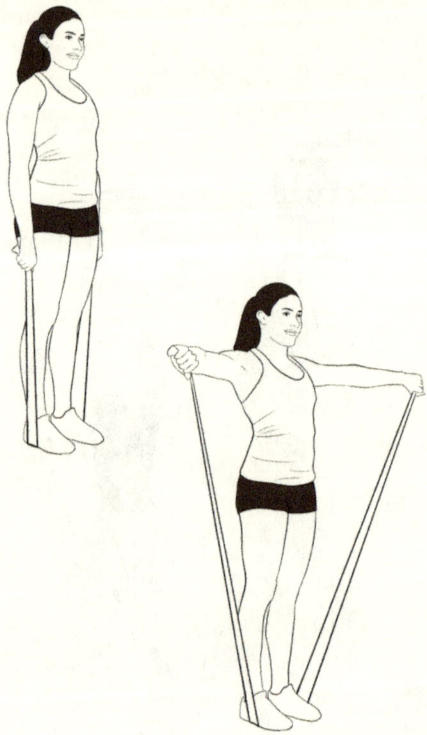

Band: Long band, either with handles, tube, or therapy band.

Step 1: Stand with a straight back, one foot or both standing over the middle of the band holding the ends of the band with both hands. Place your arms by your side, straight, and palms facing in towards your body.

Step 2: With a slight bend in your elbows, lift your arms to the side until they are shoulder height. Return to the original position.

Beginner: Use just your bodyweight or a lighter band.

Advanced: Use a stronger band or hold the band closer to the middle.

21.) Upright row

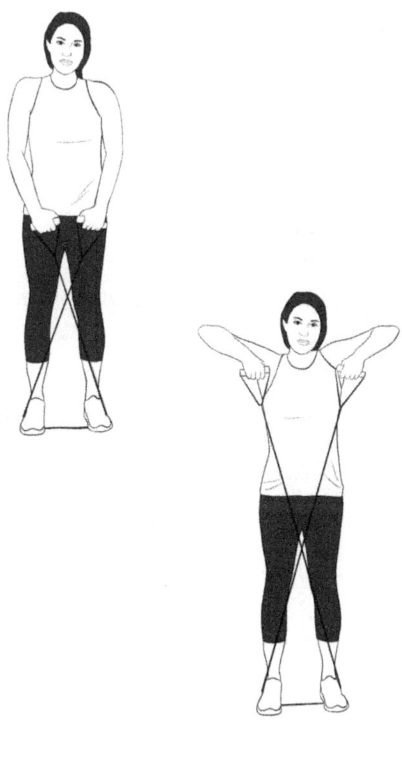

Band: Long band, either with handles, a tube, or a therapy band.

Step 1: Stand with a straight back and feet shoulder-width apart over the middle of the band. Cross the band once in front of your body and hold the ends of the band with both hands, palms facing towards you.

Step 2: Bend at the elbow and keep your palms facing you and reach your elbows to the sides and your palms towards your chest. Return to the original position.

Beginner: Use just your bodyweight or a lighter band.

Advanced: Use a stronger band or hold the band closer to the middle.

22.) Overhead pull apart

Band: Medium-sized band, either looped, with handles, a tube, or a therapy band.

Step 1: Stand with feet shoulder-width apart and a straight back, holding the ends of the band in both hands. Extend your arms above your head with straight elbows, palms facing away from your body.

Step 2: Reach your arms to opposite sides of the room, stopping at shoulder height, then return to the original position.

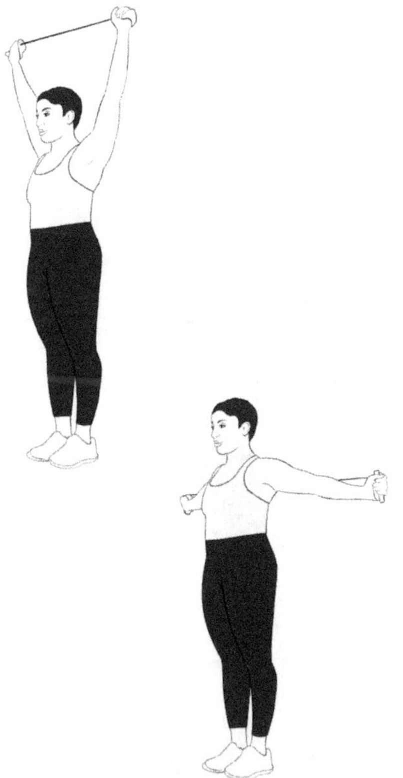

Beginner: Use just your bodyweight or a lighter band. Modify to sit.

Advanced: Use a stronger band or hold closer to the middle.

BACK

23.) Rows

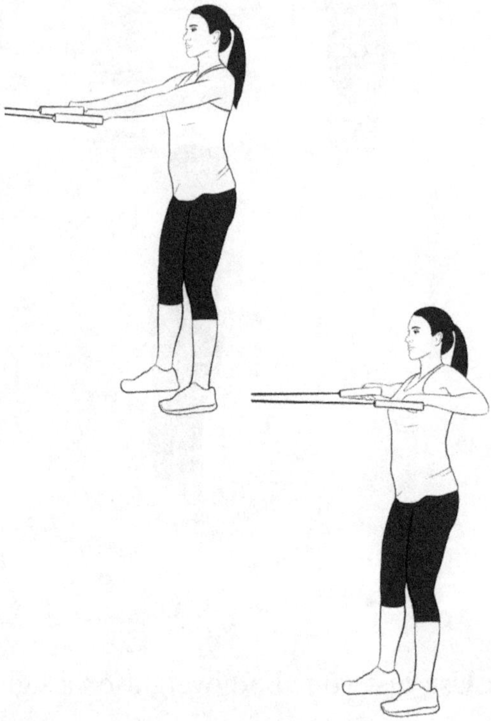

Band: Requires a medium to long band, either with handles, a tube, or a therapy band.

Step 1: Anchor the middle of the band to a stable object like a doorframe, holding the ends of the band with both hands, palms facing towards your body, and shoulder-width apart.

Step 2: Bend at the elbows and pull your palms towards your torso, then return to the original position.

Beginner: Use just your bodyweight or a lighter band. Move closer to the anchor for less resistance. Modify to sit.

Advanced: Use a stronger band or move further from the anchor.

24.) Lat pulldown

Band: Medium-sized band, either with handles, a tube, or a therapy band.

Step 1: Standing with a straight back and your feet shoulder-width apart, hold the ends of the band with both hands. Extend your arms above your head, palms facing forward.

Step 2: Bend one elbow to reach your elbow to the ribcage, directly side. Return to the original position.

Beginner: Use just your bodyweight or a lighter band.

Advanced: Use a stronger band or hold closer to the middle of the band.

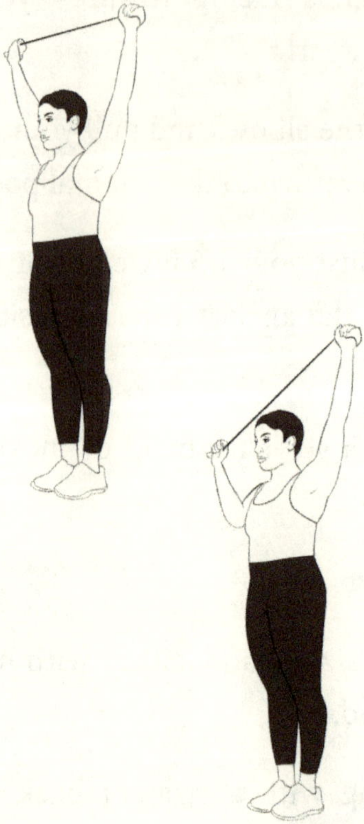

25.) Pull apart

Band: Medium to long band, either with handles, a tube, or a therapy band.

Step 1: Standing with a straight back and your feet shoulder-width apart, hold the ends of the band with both hands. Extend your arms to the front, parallel to the floor, palms facing down.

Step 2: Pull the band in opposite directions by reaching your arms to the sides. Return to the original position.

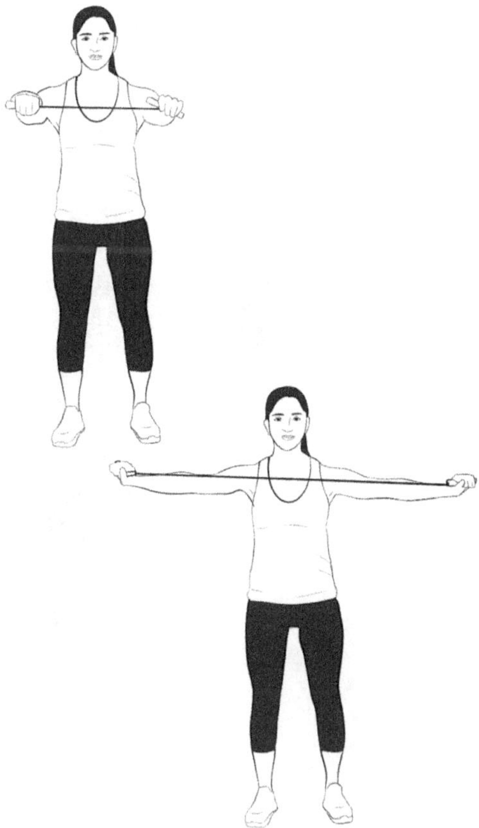

Beginner: Use just your bodyweight, a lighter band, or don't open your arms all the way. Modify to sit.

Advanced: Use a stronger band or hold closer to the middle of the band.

26.) Rear delt pull

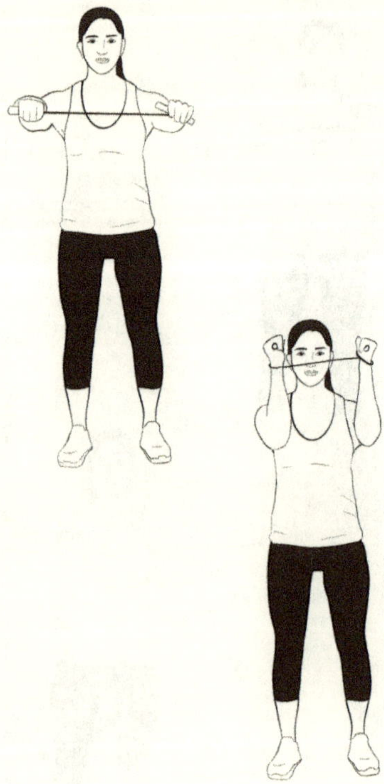

Band: Short band, either looped or therapy band looped.

Step 1: Tie the band together to create a loop that both your arms can fit through. Place the loop around both wrists, and extend your arms to the front, parallel to the floor, palms facing down.

Step 2: Bend your elbows to create a 90-degree angle, shoulders in line with your elbows, then return to the original position.

Beginner: Use a larger loop to create less resistance.

Advanced: Use a smaller loop for more resistance.

27.) Banded deadlift

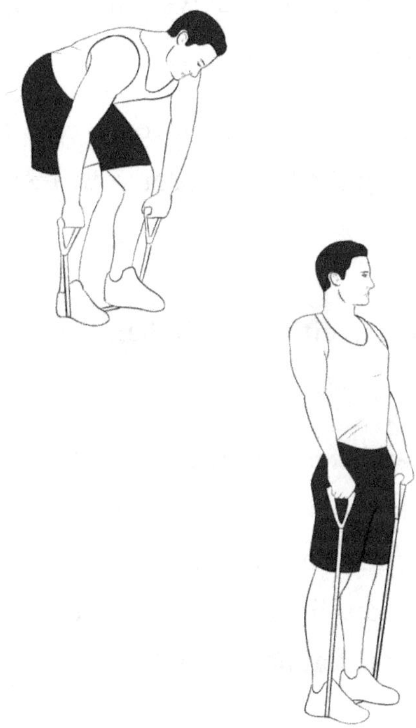

Band: Medium to long band, either with handles, a tube, or a therapy band.

Step 1: Stand with a straight back and feet shoulder-width apart over the middle of the band holding the ends of the band in both hands.

Step 2: Bend at the hips to lean forward with a slight bend at the knees and a flat back. Return to the starting position.

Beginner: Use just your bodyweight or a lighter band. Only bend forward slightly.

Advanced: Use a stronger band or create more resistance by stretching the band under your feet.

28.) Bent over rows

Band: Long band, either with handles, a tube, or a therapy band.

Step 1: Stand with feet shoulder-width apart over the middle of the band. Hold the ends of the band in both hands with extended arms straight down, palms facing towards your body. Bend at the hips to create a diagonal line with your flat back. Slightly bend at the knees.

Step 2: Bend your elbows, while holding them close to your torso, and bring your hands to your chest, then return to the original position.

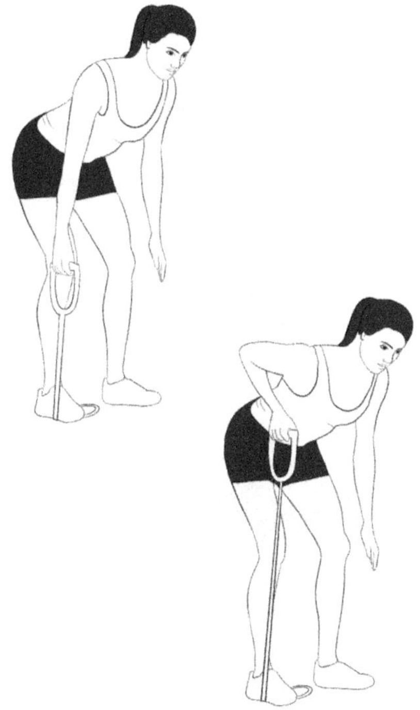

Beginner: Use a lighter band. Alternate arms instead of doing both at the same time.

Advanced: Use a stronger band.

CORE

29.) Kneeling crunch

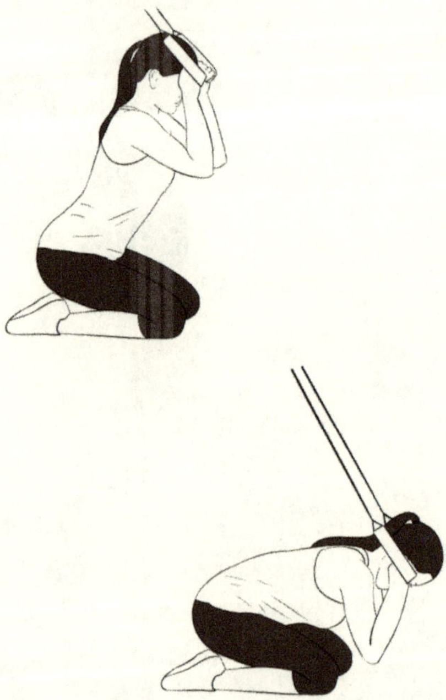

Band: Long band, either a tube or therapy band.

Step 1: Anchor the band to a stable support like the top of a door frame. Kneel on the ground with your back to the anchor while holding the band over the shoulder, palms at your shoulders, and elbows held close to the torso. Keep your hips lifted off your feet.

Step 2: Bend at the hips so that you lean forward with a straight back, and return to the original position.

Beginner: Don't bend as low. Place a pillow or mat under your knees.

Advanced: Bend so that you come closer to the ground.

30.) Resistance bicycle

Band: Short to medium-sized band, either looped, a tube, or therapy band looped.

Step 1: Tie the band together to create a loop that both your feet can fit through. Laying on your back, place the band around your feet and create a 90-degree angle with your legs by bending your knees. Lift your chin to your chest so that your shoulder blades come off the floor with your arms behind your head.

Step 2: Reach one elbow to the opposite knee, and extend the other leg then switch sides so that you create a bicycle motion with your legs.

Beginner: Use just your bodyweight or a larger loop.

Advanced: Use a stronger band or a smaller loop. Try to touch your elbow to knee.

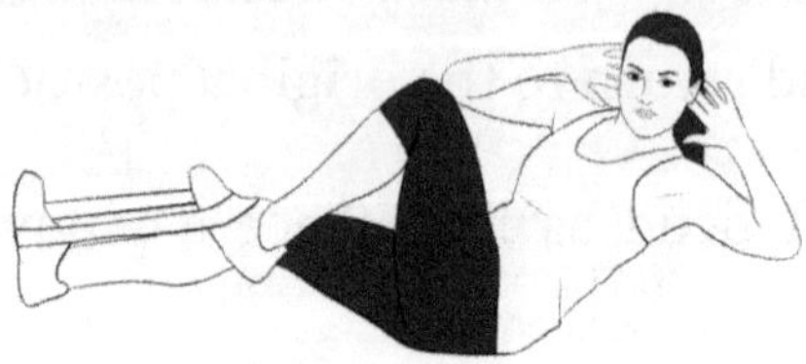

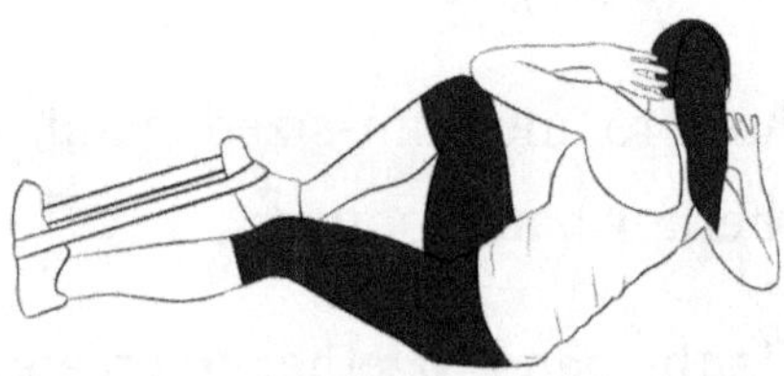

31.) Woodchopper

Band: Long band, either with handles, a tube, or a therapy band.

Step 1: Anchor one side of the band around a stable support like a heavy chair about ankle height off the floor. Standing side-by-side to the anchor, hold the band in both hands with a straight back and feet shoulder-width apart, arms extended towards the anchor.

Step 2: Pull your arms diagonally across and up your body while keeping your arms extended. Slightly pivot the hip closest to the anchor to support the movement and twist the torso and shoulders. Return to the original position.

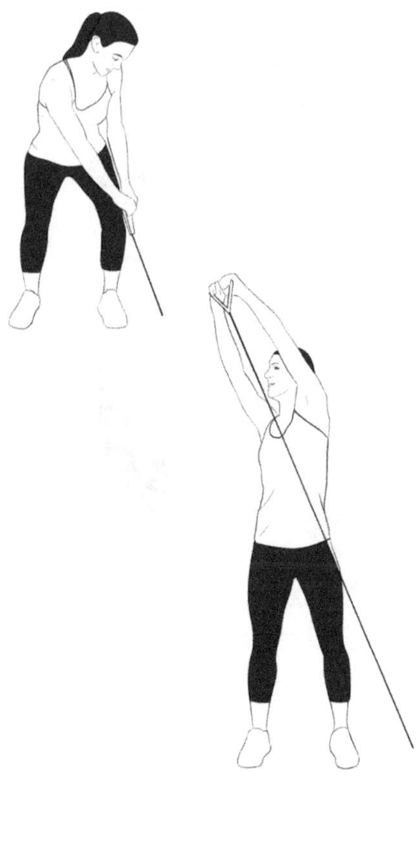

Beginner: Use just your bodyweight or mover closer to the anchor.

Advanced: Move further from the anchor or place your hands closer to the middle of the band.

32.) Reverse crunch

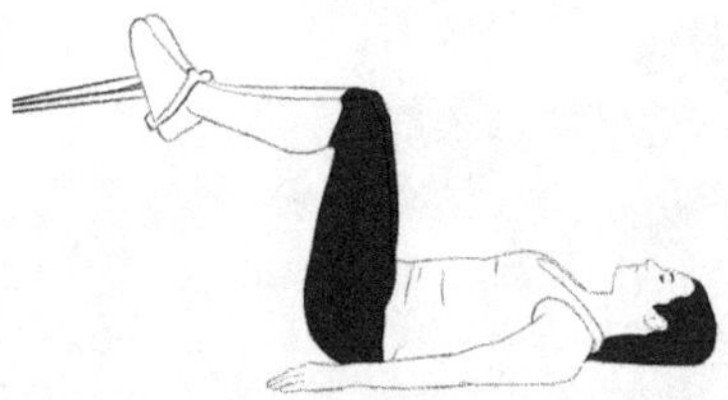

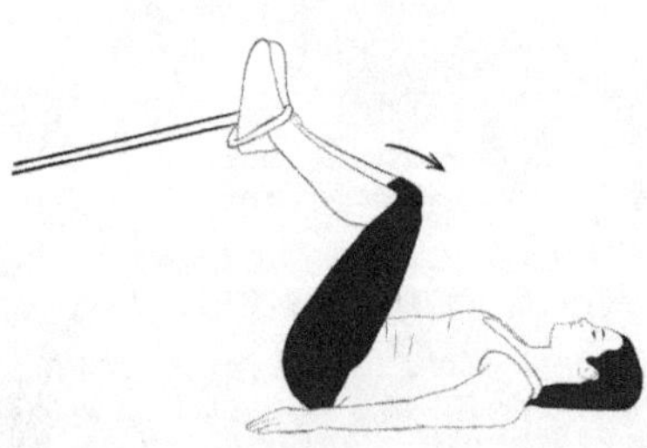

Band: Medium-sized band, either looped, or a therapy band looped.

Step 1: Tie the band together to create a loop that both your feet can fit through. Anchor the band around a stable object like a chair slightly off the ground and loop the band around your feet while laying on your back with your legs at a 90-degree angle off the ground, bent at the knees.

Step 2: Curl your lower back to bring your knees to your chest and lift your hips off the ground. Return to the original position.

Beginner: Use just your bodyweight or move closer to the anchor.

Advanced: Use a stronger band or move further from the anchor. Lift your chin to chest and shoulder blades off the floor.

33.) Resistance Russian twists

Band: Short to medium-sized band, either looped, with handles, or a therapy band.

Step 1: Sit on the floor with your legs in front and slightly bent with your feet on the floor, wrap the band around the underside of your feet and hold the ends of the band with both hands. Slightly lean backward, holding a straight back.

Step 2: Twist your torso and shoulders to one side by bringing your hands to one hip and bring everything back to the center, towards the other side, and repeat.

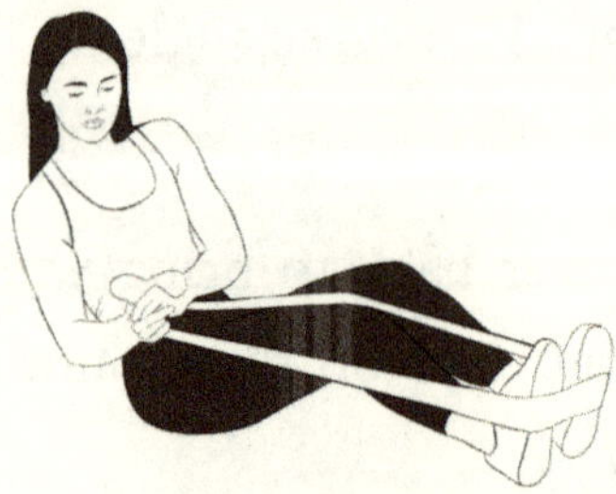

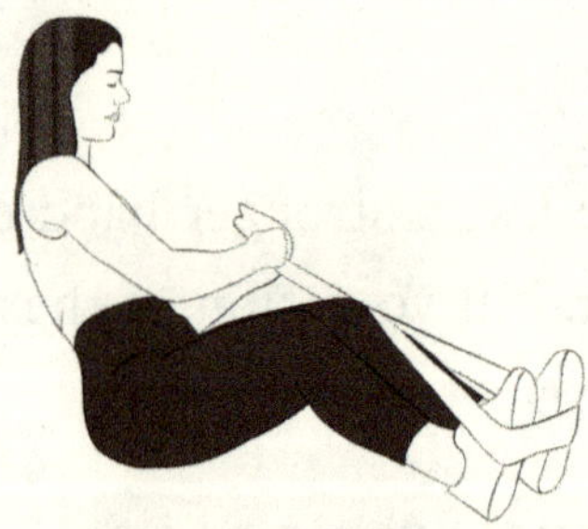

Beginner: Use just your bodyweight. Don't lean as far back.

Advanced: Use a stronger or shorter band. Lift your feet off the ground into a tabletop position.

34.) Leg lowers

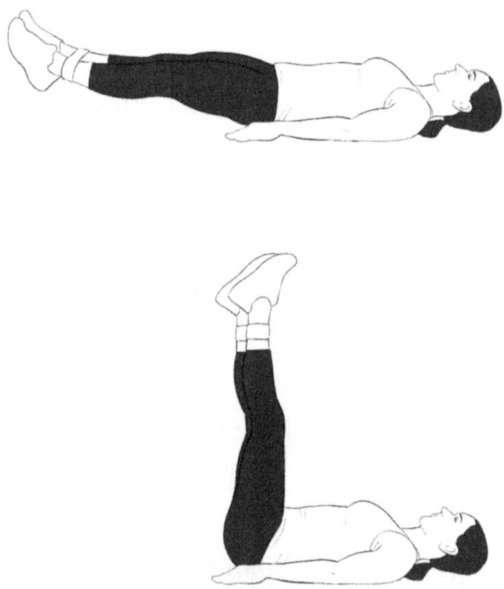

Band: Short band, either looped or a therapy band looped.

Step 1: Tie the band together to create a loop that both your feet can fit through. Loop the band above the ankles and separate your legs to shoulder-width apart.

Step 2: Laying on your back, bring your legs up towards the ceiling to create a 90-degree angle at your hips. Think about reaching your navel to your spine to activate your abdominal muscles as you lower your legs without losing the activation. Return to the original position.

Beginner: Only lower your legs about a foot below the starting position.

Advanced: Lower your legs, so they are only a few inches to a foot off the ground.

FULL BODY

35.) Squat to adduction

Band: Short to medium-sized band, either looped or a therapy band looped.

Step 1: Tie the band together to create a loop that both your legs can fit through. Loop the band below the knees. Standing with feet shoulder-width apart and a straight back, bend your knees and slightly lean forward as if you were about to sit in a chair.

Step 2: Straighten your knees and back into a neutral position as you shift your weight to one side, lifting the opposite foot out to the side. Return to the original position.

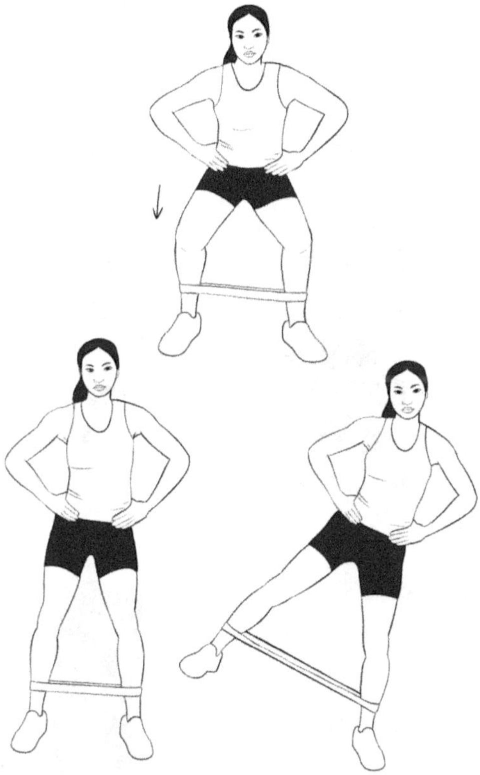

Beginner: Use a larger loop. Don't squat too low, and lift your leg three to five inches off the ground. Hold onto an anchor for support.

Advanced: Use a smaller loop. Try to fully squat and lift your leg about a foot off the ground.

36.) Squat to overhead press

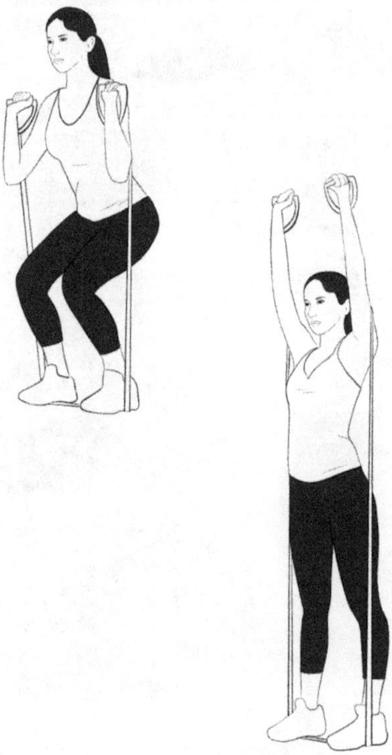

Band: Long band, either with handles, a tube, or a therapy band.

Step 1: Standing on the middle of the band with feet shoulder-width apart, hold the ends of the band with both hands. Place your hands on top of your shoulders, elbows pointed forward, and palms up. Bend your knees and slightly lean forward as if you were about to sit in a chair.

Step 2: Straighten your knees and back into a neutral position as you extend your arms overhead, then lower down into the original squatting position.

Beginner: Don't squat too low. Use a lighter band or just your bodyweight.

Advanced: Try to squat fully. Use a stronger band or hold the band closer to the middle.

37.) Band side step

Band: Short band, either looped or a therapy band looped.

Step 1: Tie the band together to create a loop that both your legs can fit through.

Step 2: Place the band above your knees, bend the knees and slightly lean forward as if you were about to sit in a chair. Holding this position, step to the side with one foot, then close the distance with the other foot, like a crab walk.

Beginner: Take smaller steps or use a larger band.

Advanced: Take larger steps or use a smaller band.

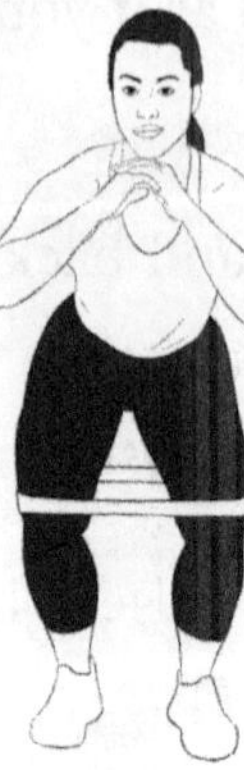

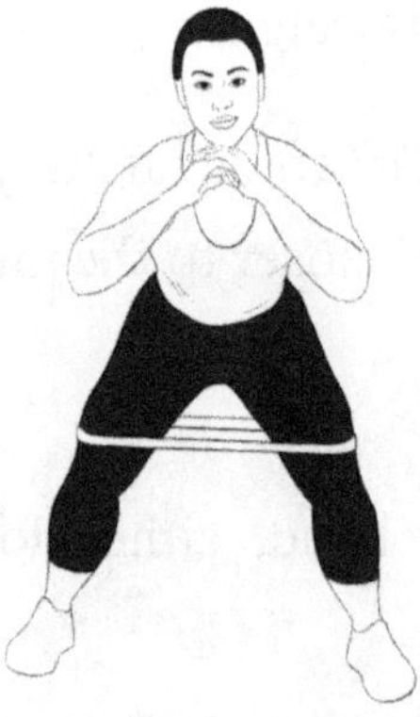

38.) Bent over row

Band: Medium-sized band, either looped, with handles, a tube, or a therapy band.

Step 1: While in a standing lunge position, place your front foot over one end of the band and hold the other end in your hand on the same side that your foot is anchoring the band. Lean forward so that your back creates a diagonal line, palm facing in towards your body.

Step 2: Pull the band towards your chest by bending the elbow and holding it close to your torso, then release and return to the original position.

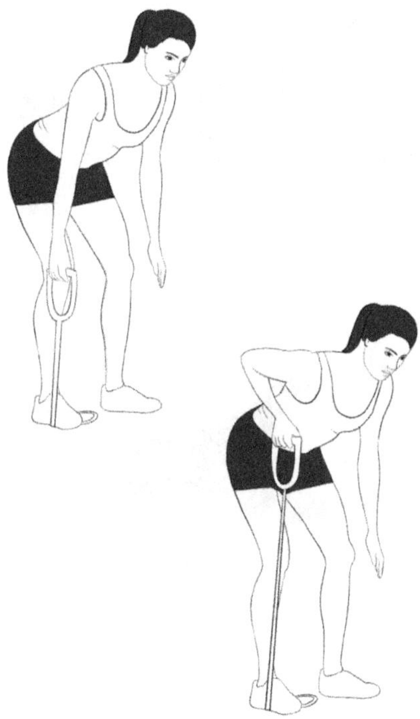

Beginner: Use just your bodyweight or a lighter band.

Advanced: Create a deeper lung by bending the front knee more. Hold the band closer to the middle.

39.) Plank banded leg lifts

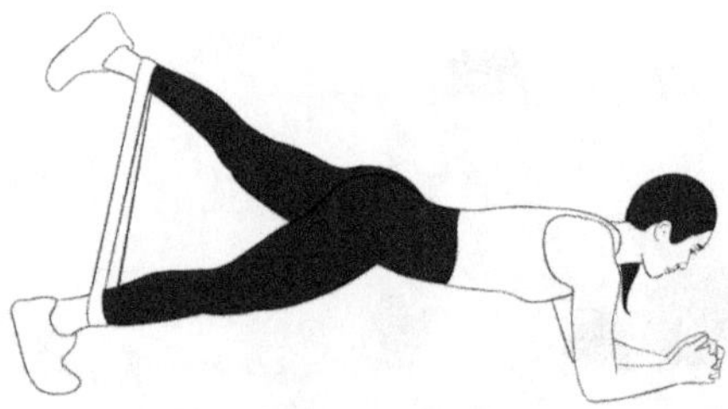

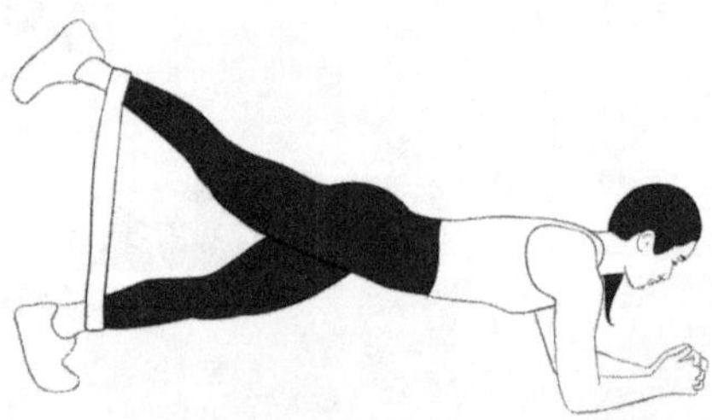

Band: Short band, either looped or a therapy band looped.

Step 1: Tie the band together to create a loop that both your legs can fit through. Loop the band above the ankles. Support yourself in a plank position by setting your hands and feet on the floor and keeping your torso straight.

Step 2: Keeping your legs straight, lift one off the floor by aiming your heel to the ceiling just a few inches off the floor. Return to the original position.

Beginner: Plank against a wall instead of on the floor. Use a larger loop.

Advanced: Plank on your elbows rather than hands. Use a smaller loop.

40.) Standing crunch

Band: Short to medium-sized band, either with handles, a tube, or a therapy band.

Step 1: Standing with a straight back and your feet shoulder-width apart, hold the ends of the band with both hands. Extend your arms in front of you parallel to the floor, palms facing down.

Step 2: Twist your torso and shoulders to one side, while holding the band tight, and lift the knee on that side to reach the middle of the band to the knee. Return to the original position.

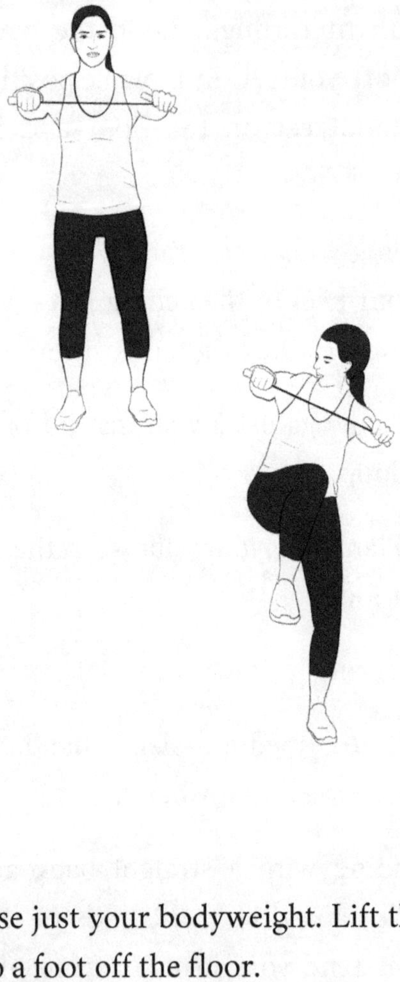

Beginner: Use just your bodyweight. Lift the leg only a few inches to a foot off the floor.

Advanced: Use a stronger band. Try to touch your hand to the opposite knee.

CONCLUSION

As a senior, you have a deep connection to your body, and know what is or isn't good for your health. The exercises are now available to you at your own convenience, and it is your choice to take the next step into a more active, convenient, and healthy lifestyle. By creating your own health or physique goals, you can use a combination of exercises found in the Arms, Legs, Chest, Shoulders, Back, Core, and Full Body segments of this guide. The number of workouts one can create with these 40 exercises alone can sustain a full, healthy body. Modifications like moving slower, holding at the height of the movement, or switching band strength and styles can also bring a new dynamic to your routine.

In the near future, when you become more comfortable and confident in your resistance band training, you have the ability to increase repetitions, sets, and band strength. On the other hand, the option to decrease the number of sets, repetitions, or band strength is your decision to make based on what you feel with your body.

Like any other type of workout style, resistance band workouts are a great way for you to maintain your physical health, and all you need is the additional support of motivation and determination. Setting clear and achievable goals will help you stay focused, and holding onto inspiration helps make any challenge easier. Maintain a strict schedule, and don't be afraid to dedicate a small corner of your house for exercising. Following the perfect pre-workout routine will help you get into the right mindset.

REFERENCES

Davis, K. (2016, January). *33 resistance band exercises you can do literally anywhere*. Greatist. Retrieved from https://greatist.com/fitness/resistance-band-exercises#legs-and-glutes

5 types of resistance bands & which are best?1. SET FOR SET. (2020, October 13). Retrieved from https://www.setforset.com/blogs/news/5-types-of-resistance-bands-which-is-best-to-buy

Harris-Fry, N. (2021, December 4). *Blast your whole body with this resistance band workout*. coachmaguk. Retrieved from https://www.coachmag.co.uk/full-body-workouts/6867/blast-your-whole-body-with-this-resistance-band-workout

Kraemer, W.J., Ratamess, N.A. & French, D.N. Resistance training for health and performance. *Curr Sports Med Rep* 1, 165–171 (2002). https://doi.org/10.1007/s11932-002-0017-7

Mansour, S. (2021, March 19). *At-home resistance band workout that improves balance, strength and flexibility.* NBCNews.com. Retrieved from https://www.nbcnews.com/select/lifestyle/one-month-resistance-band-workout-you-can-do-anywhere-ncna965461

Schmitz, D. (2019, December 17). *9 reasons why aging high profile NFL athletes choose RBT*. Resistance Band Training. Retrieved from https://resistancebandtraining.com/9-reasons-aging-nfl-athletes-choose-rbt/

www.ingramcontent.com/pod-product-compliance
Lightning Source LLC
Chambersburg PA
CBHW032153020426
42334CB00016B/1270
* 9 7 8 0 6 4 5 4 2 5 8 4 0 *